Grandma's Natural Remedies And Ancient Recipes - Volume 3

How to cure a common cold and other health related remedies

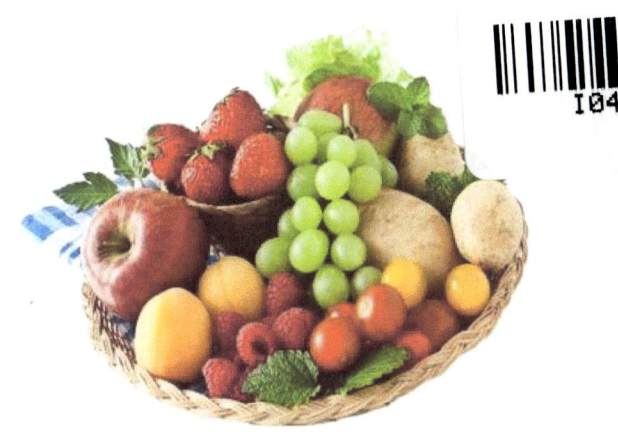

Dueep Jyot Singh

Natural Remedy Series

Mendon Cottage Books

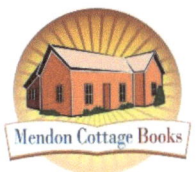

JD-Biz Publishing

Our books are available at

1. Amazon.com

2. Barnes and Noble

3. Itunes

4. Kobo

5. Smashwords

6. Google Play Books

Table of Contents

Introduction

In volume 3 of Grandma's Natural Remedies And Ancient Recipes, you are going to get to know more about a number of different fruits, and vegetables which are going to enhance your health, and allow you to live long and prosper. These natural remedies have come down through word-of-mouth from grandmother to granddaughter, down the millenniums, in almost all the ancient civilizations, when it was the responsibility of the female of the family to make sure that her family kept healthy and survived in the times when superstition and bad hygiene was rife.

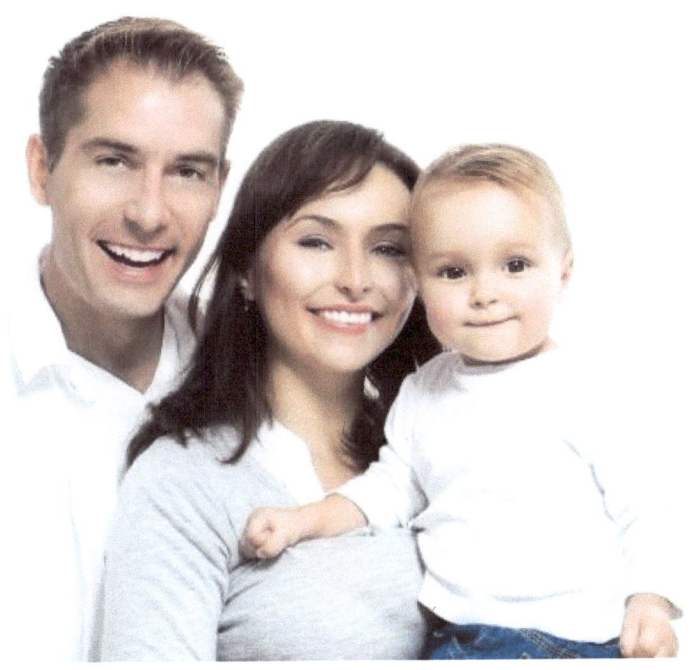

Keep your family healthy the natural way

This is the reason why so many ancient remedies and herbal recipes, were used on a day to day basis, by grandma and these volumes comprise of a collection of the wisdom of the ages for all those people who believe in the power of nature to cure ailments from the root, instead of looking for chemical-based drugs to help cure them.

Remember that those were the days, when ignorance was also rife and many quacks came up with nostrums potions and Brews. One can read about the most famous of them all, the witches brew in MacBeth . Grandma is not going to be putting eyes of newt and tongues of frogs in her remedies, but is going to tell us about how simple fruit juices and spices, can heal and cure common remedies.

Grandma knew all about how to remain beautiful, even when she was in her 80s and 90s. That is because she used the wisdom of ages, passed down to her, in simple rules of living.

Grandma's Rules For Simple Living

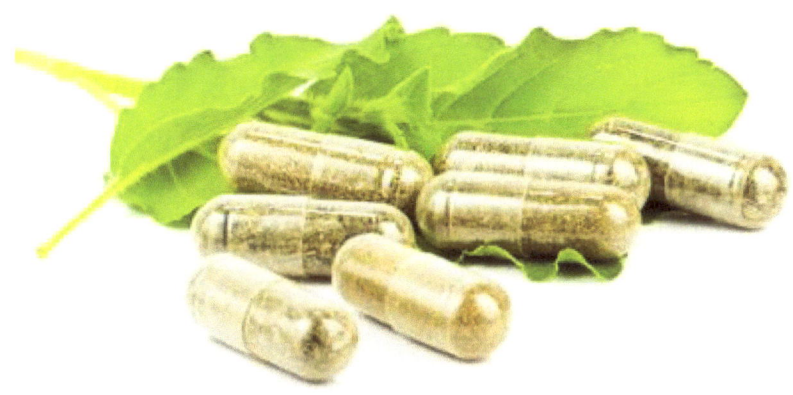

Grandma preferred natural to chemical

Here are some of her rules passed down to you and which can be easily incorporated in your own lifestyle right now.

Eat food whenever you are feeling hungry. Remember to eat 4 meals a day. Do not skip any meals, because that is going to cause you to gain weight. Eat a little less than what your hunger demands.

Do not eat too spicy and fatty foods, because these are going to interfere with your digestive system.

Remember to add salads, green and leafy vegetables, milk, yogurt, and fruit in small quantities to your daily meal and diet.

I do not know whether this is going to be helpful in a time when we use so many pesticides on our fruit and vegetables, but grandma ate fruit with the skins and peels on, especially citrus fruit.

She was also very fond of sprouted beans, especially mung sprouts. This was mixed with lemons, tomatoes, green chilies and a little bit of rock salt to give the extra spicy Tang and taste to a healthy food accompaniment.

Look in all the ancient and medieval recipes of cookery – Egyptian, Persian, Elizabethan, Spanish, and any other civilization or era you like. You are going to notice that all of the food is either broiled or baked or roasted. Frying, grilling, and even roasting removes most of the beneficial ingredients and nutrients in food. The ancients advocated you to eat food in its natural state, which means raw after you had washed it well. But then at that time, the air, water and atmosphere was not contaminated heavily with chemical pollutants.

Alas, we cannot eat food in its natural state, because we are going to be encouraging toxins in our bodies. So one would suggest looking for organically grown plants, with just the bare minimum of chemical fertilizers, sprinkled on them to get rid of pests.

In the East, a mixture of tobacco water and Neem seed extract water solution is sprinkled on the plants to get rid of pests naturally. This has been done in the East through millenniums, however much some people consider this to be a relatively modern 19th and 20th century "discovery."

Money oriented chemical Fertilizer companies want to prove that this is definitely not a workable solution, but it has worked for millenniums in the

East, thus ensuring that our ancestors did not ingest potentially fatal poisons, with every bite of fruit and vegetables, they ate.

Grandma used a few crystals of potassium permanganate added to the water to wash fruits and vegetables and get rid of any insects. This also got rid of all particles of dust and dirt.

Grandma encouraged her family to fast one day a week. Now for everybody who is under the impression that the word "fast" means not eating anything throughout the day, and this thought in itself is anathema to most of us will enjoy our food, real fasting is quite something different.

You are going to eat lemons and other citrus fruit, fresh fruit, salads, buttermilk and nuts throughout the day. No tea or coffee. The idea is to detoxify your body, and get rid of all the extra toxins accumulated during the week when you have been eating lots of fatty, greasy, fried, and hard to digest junk food.

This practice is still in Vogue in many parts of the East. Fill up a copper kettle or utensil with water and leave it overnight. Drink two glasses of this water 1st thing in the morning. It is going to clear up your system. It is also going to make sure that any sort of copper deficiency in your body is supplemented and renewed with copper ions every day. This also helps in eliminating accumulated toxins collected in your body. Try it out.

Do not drink tea first thing in the morning. You may have fruit juice for breakfast. Do not go to work on an empty stomach, just because you are missing your train connection to the city. I remember one of my busy busy busy police officer friends saying, "I never get out of my house, without having a good breakfast, because one never knows when I will have the time to have another meal." This is quite a good citation, because the ham/bacon with hot buttered toast and fried eggs enjoyed with fresh fruit juice breakfast gives him so much energy, that he is considered a dynamo in his department.

Alas, most of us do not consider ourselves properly awake until we can reach for a cup of hot coffee and get our caffeine boost. You may not know it, but your body is addicted to caffeine. Try reducing your caffeine intake. You are going to find yourself sleeping better and even healthier.

In ancient times, the sages suggested that water not be drunk with meals. That would facilitate the mixing of the saliva in the mouth with every mouthful chewed properly. They also spoke about chewing your mouthful in such a manner, that it was more of a liquid than a solid mouthful. If you really wanted to drink some water, just because the food was too spicy, you could have a couple of sips. Or you could alleviate the burning sensation on your tongue, with some cooling yogurt.

Those sages ate yogurt with every meal, and also drank buttermilk in huge quantities. This buttermilk was lightly flavored with rock salt and dried roasted powdered cumin which is an excellent digestive spice. If you really wanted to drink water, you drank it half an hour before and after meals. The liquid intake during your meal could be supplemented with buttermilk, yogurt, juice, fruit, and anything else easily digestible, natural and liquid.

The ancients worked hard outdoors from dawn to dusk. Unfortunately, we have forgotten the idea of physical labor, and that is why we spend so much time in our gyms trying desperately hard to get back into shape. Blame our sedentary lifestyles for this, gym -based exercise duty lifestyle.

So if you can manage to get a little swimming and some walking done throughout the day, which is enough to tone up some of the muscles in your body. This exercise is also enough to give you a good appetite for a good, healthy meal.

Believe it or not, gardening is also an excellent way to keep healthy. You manage to do some constructive work outdoors, move from place to place, and exercise your body while weeding, routing, pruning, planting and doing other outdoor gardening activities.

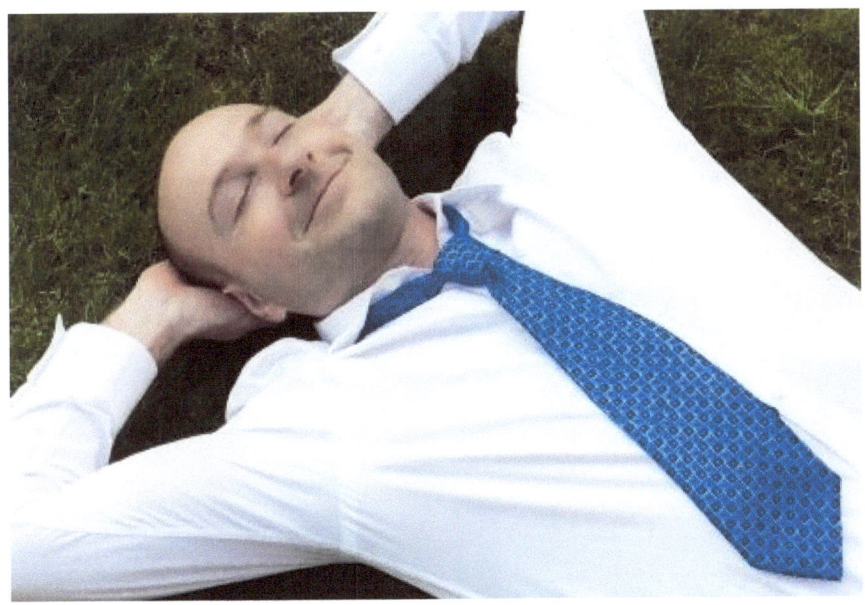

Get into the habit of walking in a garden, breathing deeply. The breathing should be done in inhale – exhale motions from the bottom of the lungs. You need to straighten up your chest to do that. Most of us breathe superficially "from the top of our lungs," because we do not want to breathe in polluted air. This reduces our lung power. Deep breathing should be done – and is most beneficial – only when you are in an area full of trees. At least here you are going to be protected from the chemical pollution in your city and the fresh oxygen is going to tone up your system.

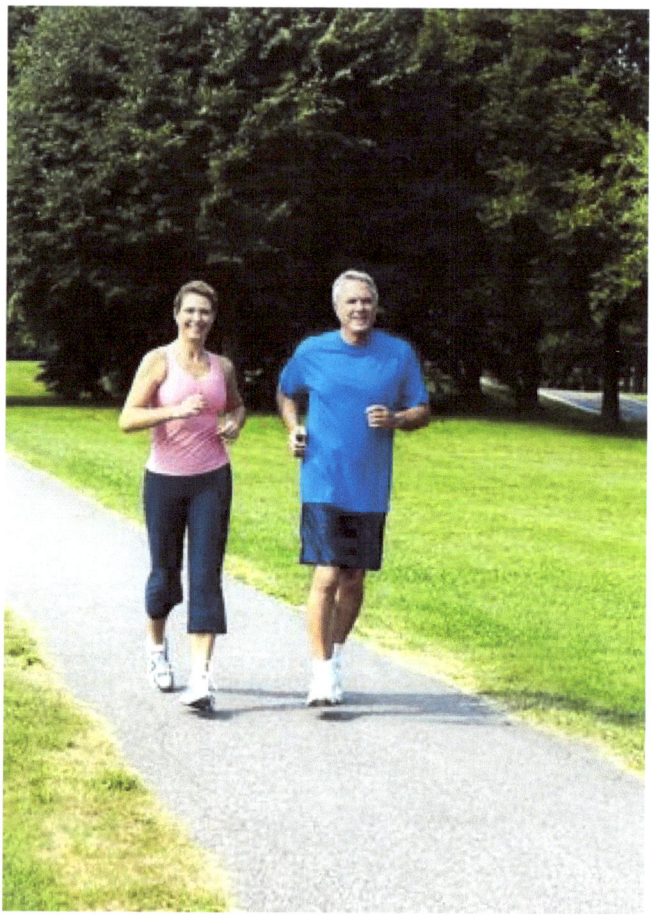

If you enjoy jogging, do that in the fresh air, at least once a day. Remember runners of ancient times who used to run the marathon. It is a well-known historical fact that the soldiers of Chaka Zulu and other African warriors had trained themselves to run 30 miles – each way – a day, and *fight a battle at the end of it*, win the battle and come back home with their trophies. Now they had style. And this was in the 19 century.

The 20th century human being has become lazy, because he has no physical challenge to challenge his mental and physical strength. Unless he is called upon to do so, he would rather sit hunched up in front of his computer, laptop, or TV and spend lots of time munching snacks out of a plastic bag.

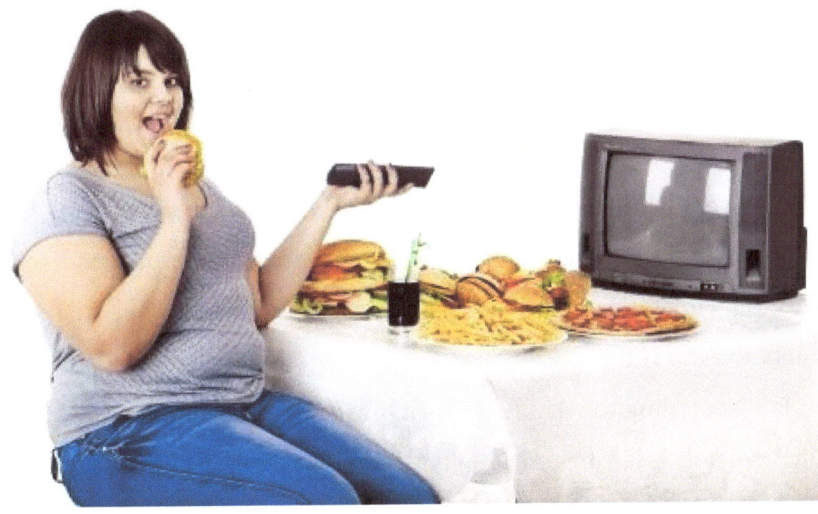

Is it any wonder why so many human beings are suffering from problems like obesity, chronic diseases and other ailments, brought about by this totally unhealthy lifestyle? The ancients had a light breakfast of sprouted grains and buttermilk. A heavy breakfast full of proteins, minerals, and carbohydrates was taken by only those people who had to do hard physical labor throughout the day.

Grandma definitely did not advocate the unlimited eating of sweetmeats for her children. Sweets were given to them in limited quantities, in the form of fudge, biscuits, puddings and other desserts, to allow them to have the necessary sugar intake needed to keep their systems moving properly. But in the 20th century, children found that their parents allowed them to eat unlimited quantities of chocolate, bubble gums, toffees, ice cream, chewing gums and even corn syrup based food items. That is why the general health of the children started to deteriorate due to this excess of sugar intake.

Along with that, believe it or not, most of the illnesses in adults and children are caused due to the intake of aerated colas and soft drinks. They have become an integral part of every social gathering. You also find them in your fridge, in the shape of diet colas and cokes. Did you know that they originally were made by a chemist, as a digestive? He suggested you drink 3 tablespoons of this cola if you are suffering from tummy problems like indigestion. However, we drink bottles of these colas whenever we feel remotely thirsty. If the Coca-Cola Company is still using the original formula – according to what it says – in the proportions written out by its original creator, it is single-handedly destroying the health of generations, without imparting a statutory warning label on their Coke bottles.

Grandma was also a firm believer in allowing her children to cook in the sun after they were massaged with olive oil or mustard oil. Greek children in ancient times went unclad in the sun, till the age of 5, because their grandmothers knew that they had to be healthy warriors and she needed to get their bodies accustomed to plenty of vitamin K. No wonder Greeks were sun worshipers, because the massaging with olive oil and sun baking promoted the muscle growth in the limbs of the children, kept them healthy, and also made them used to exercising outdoors in the form of play. Unfortunately, moms nowadays will rather have their kiddies stay indoors, because the sun would harm. They dedicate complexions, would not it. Also, the idea of their playing outdoors in all seasons is horrors, not to be thought of at all. This is the reason why such a large number of children have weak muscle tone, hate the idea of exercise and also have poor autoimmune systems, because cooped up in a stuffy atmosphere in their houses prevent them from growing healthy, naturally.

Never have a bath immediately after you have had a meal. Some of us have the habit of having a shower before we go to sleep to get rid of all the stress and strain and grime of a hard day. But that is about 2 hours after we have had our meal, and we are ready to go to sleep now. Remember, do not go straight up to bed, after you have had a heavy meal. Your stomach is definitely not going to thank you for the burden placed on it to digest that meal, when you and your brain are in shutdown for sleep mode.

So now that you know all about grandma's ideas and views about how to keep healthy, incorporating these ideas into your lifestyle right now may change drastically into a   healthier, calm and stress-free you.

Grandma's Easy Health Remedies

Wake Up Energy Drink

You may want to wake up to this tasty wake up remedy, which keeps you fresh, healthy and energetic throughout the day. Soak 4 almonds and 4 raisins along with 4 peppercorns in water overnight. Then make a paste of it in the morning and drink this down with a glass of warm milk. This has been an integral part of many eastern breakfasts for centuries.

Grandma knew that prevention was better than cure, and that is why she knew that most of her kids would suffer from skin diseases one time or the other in their lives. That was because the water sources could easily get contaminated, and thus cause skin ailments to breakout on the once smooth skins of her childrens' bodies.

In ancient times, common people did not have specially made bathrooms in which they could clean themselves, so they took a dip in the nearby river and pond, especially in the summer. The livestock of the village also considered the pond to be an easily accessible drinking and bathing ground. So grandma tried her own natural health remedies to prevent the skin outbreaks.

She often asked her family members to wash in a solution made up of half a rind of lemon, some rose petals and some Neem leaves. After 20 minutes she told them to go ahead and have a bath in any water source, contaminated or uncontaminated. In the 21th century, I continue this skin purifying procedure by just placing these ingredients in a bucket full of water, and then pour that water over myself, 20 minutes later.

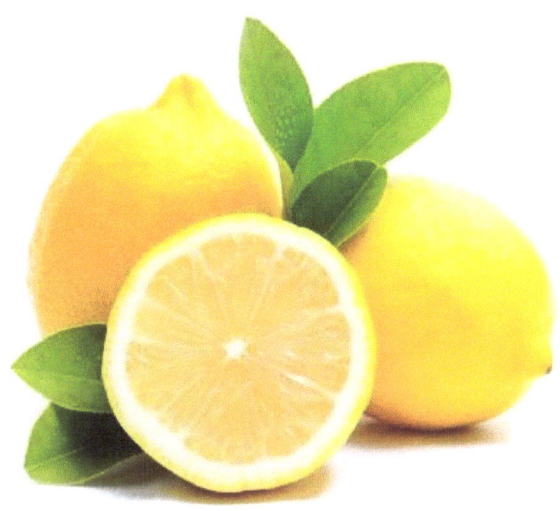

Lemon is an extremely good astringent. It also prevents body odor, especially in the summer. The rose is just to give the exotic fragrance of roses to a bath, making that activity a pleasure instead of a boring duty! The Neem leaves are considered to be one of the best natural antiseptics to prevent skin diseases in any form or shape since ancient times.

Benefits of the Neem [Azadirachta Indica]

Do not have a Neem plant growing in your garden? Ask your nearest nursery owner to get one for you. This plant is an air purifier. Its seeds can be used as organic fertilizer and a natural pesticide. Its leaves can be used to prevent skin ailments, especially pimples. Neem oil extract should be worth its weight in gold, because a few drops of Neem oil keeps your skin healthy, your mouth fresh, when used as a mouthwash, and when added to your shampoo is going to prevent scalp diseases, including dandruff or eczema.

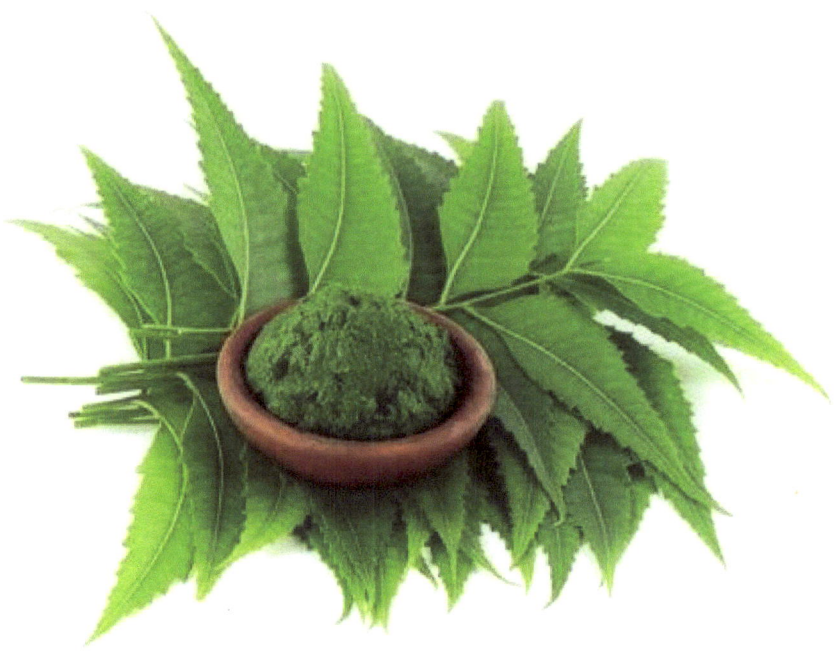

Neem can be grown almost anywhere, because it is an extremely hardy plant. In ancient India, there was the belief that the God of death did not enter very often, in a house which had a Neem plant growing in it. Perhaps this was the way to say that every single part of the Neem plant was used to keep the inmates of the house healthy. That is why people buying houses in India, ask just one question – is there a Neem plant in the garden? How far is the nearest Neem? This plant was also worshiped in ancient times with the idea that friendly spirits lived on it, and blessed the house in which they were allowed to flourish undisturbed.

Curing a Cold

Tasty Cold Whisky Remedy

This was given to me by a Scottish friend, and naturally, it would have the water of life in it. Anyway, this remedy is for all those people who have access to a whiskey bottle nearby and do not mind dosing themselves with something to feed the cold. Dougal told me that he used to be miserable whenever he caught a cold, but now he does not mind it, because he is curing himself with this remedy. Do not try it out on children and babies!

25 g of rock candy – [crystallized sugar]; one pint your favorite whiskey, one pint of water; 1 teaspoon glycerin ; half a teaspoon of lemon juice – mix all together; this is automatically going to become a syrup. Take one teaspoonful as often as required. This is an excellent cold cure remedy.

Well, I remember being dosed with one spoonful of brandy by my grandmother, followed by hot milk to prevent colds in the winter. The cold disappeared – or never appeared – but at 8 o'clock sharp, every evening, I would begin to cough and honk and sniff, because I wanted a spoonful of that tasty warming delicious brandy, out of grandpa's medicine/brandy closet. I was 25 at that time, and am a total teetotaler, so I guess that was the only time when a nondrinking adult got addicted to A Spoonful of Brandy Makes the Winter More Bearable!

Butter Cold Syrup

Take one-half cup of molasses, half a teaspoonful of butter and one tablespoon vinegar. Boil together and put it in a glass bottle. Give the patient one teaspoonful or less as the case requires and as often as possible, until the patient is cured. This can be given to children.

Gingered Lemon Drink

Try drinking ginger juice with lemon and hot water. This is a surefire recipe for preventing and curing colds. 2 spoons full of ginger juice and 1 spoonful of lemon in one glass of hot water. Allow the patient to sip it slowly. This is going to prevent him from being dehydrated. Well, since ancient times lemon juice was used to prevent colds in the winter, but now we know that vitamin C is the main ingredient in citric fruits, which keeps you healthy. So instead of eating vitamin C tablets, drink lemon juice, and lots of it in warm water in the winter.

You may also want to try half a teaspoon of lemon juice and ¼ teaspoon ginger juice in one teaspoonful of honey 3 – 4 times a day. This prevents your throat from getting dry and also clears up the cough. Children love it.

In fact, the moment I began to show symptoms of a cold, after coming back from a muggy atmosphere in the office and exposure to the cold outside, I was immediately put on to a hot water lemon juice diet, with my feet placed in a master bath. That prevented the cold from developing.

Mustard Bath Powder

She made a mustard bath powder, by mixing up 8 teaspoons of baking soda with 3 tablespoons mustard powder in hot water. She added a few drops of eucalyptus essential oil to this mixture. This is a very popular British cold preventive remedy, which she brought back from Britain [she was a nurse – Lieut. in the British Army during the 2nd World War.]

I modified this mustard bath recipe by adding 2 drops of rosemary and one drop of oil of Wintergreen to this mixture, because, well, I love essential oils, which smell so delightful!

Soak your feet in this mustard bath while you are drinking lemon juice. Cover yourself up with a shawl. You may want to drink hot milk before you go to sleep, tuck yourself up in with a hot water bottle after a meal of hot chicken soup. Goodbye, colds, by the next morning. Of course, you are going to sweat like the dickens, but this balances the effect of the cold, and brings your body back to proper natural "harmony."

Why do not people try it out, more often instead of allowing the colds to continue for 3 to 4 nasty, clogged noses and heavy head days?

Hot and Cold Water Remedy

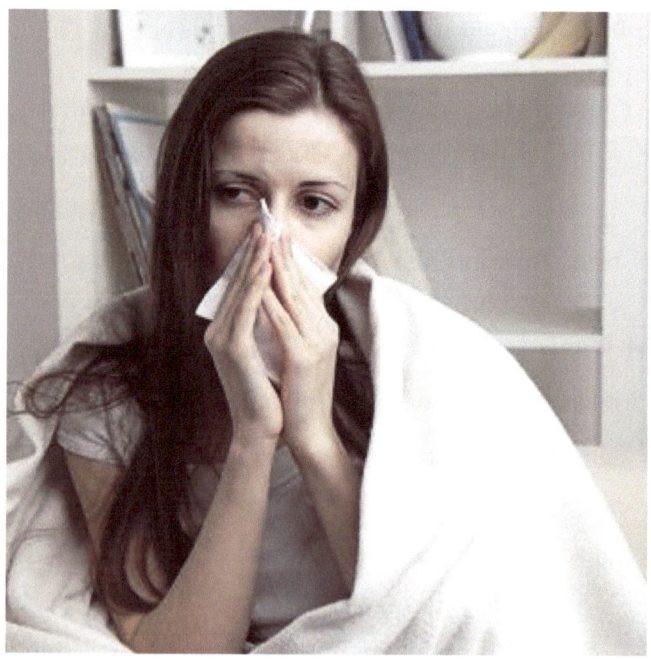

Grandma also had another very effective cold remedy where I needed to soak my feet in hot water, and drink cold water at the beginning of a cold.

Well, it may have been effective for her, but I am a pampered brat. I was not drinking cold water in the cold weather, when I had come out of the cold. You may want to try it, if you are adventurous. This is supposed to be guaranteed effective.

Traditional Chicken Soup Remedy – The Way Grandma Made It

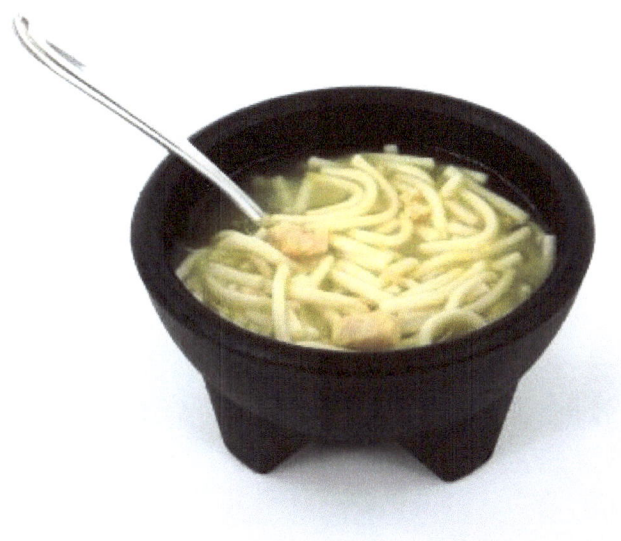

Believe it or not, chicken soup is considered to be the best soul food, apart from it being a really healthy and rejuvenating nourishing food.

Make chicken soup stock for the whole winter by taking one chicken, putting in some onion and carrots, and any other seasonal vegetables available, seasoning – the herbs used can be parsley, celery, thyme, ginger, and even a clove of garlic – and salt.

Allow it to boil till the three – four glasses of water become one glass of thick soup concentrate. She preserved this stock in a cool place in her cellar, I preserve it by placing it in an ice tray in my refrigerator. Whenever I want hot chicken soup, I just pop out two concentrate chicken cubes, add water and milk and noodles if I want to give the family chicken noodle soup, and so I am assured that they have something warm and health giving in their tummies. The chicken soup can be served with slivers of boiled chicken in it.

What about the vegetables in the chicken stock? Just remove them, dice them and toss with some olive oil. You can add seasoning and salt and pepper, and eat them as a salad or as an accompaniment? After all, all their essential nutrients have gone into the making of the chicken stock. You may also want to fry them on a griddle with just a little hint of powdered cumin seed and rocksalt. Nice and tasty.

One of my chef friends showed me a good way to see whether the noodles were cooked properly or not. Pick up a noodle and aim at the nearest kitchen wall with it. If it is cooked, it is going to stick to the wall. If it is not cooked, it is going to fall down in some place behind your cooking range, where it is going to be out of sight out of mind and not to be discovered until the next thorough spring cleaning of your kitchen! Talk about Cordon Bleu-it!

Time-tested Chest Rub

Grandma also made a chest rub for colds and congested chests. She used pork lard, and I think that is what makes these chest rubs so oily and greasy. Nevertheless, they are one-time remedies, and extremely effective.

Melt half a cup of pork lard/mutton tallow in a pan. Add 1 ½ teaspoonful of turpentine, and half a teaspoonful of red chili powder to this melted lard. I made this recipe a little strong, because I had some eucalyptus essential oil going spare. Add 2 drops of eucalyptus essential oil to this mixture. Place it in a glass bottle. Use this as a chest rub, for congested adult chests.

The chilies are going to sting a little, when they touch your skin, but they have an immediate heating affect. I also use this chest rub on the sides of my forehead, whenever I have a cold induced headache. I then cover it up with a flannel and go off to sleep assured that it is cold, cold gone away by the time I wake up the next morning.

Vaseline – Camphor Remedy

If you have Vaseline ready at hand, add a little bit of camphor to it and make it into a paste. I normally make this Vaseline – camphor mixture, right at the beginning of the winter, and place it in an easily accessible place, right next to my bed. The moment I start sniffling, I rub it inside my nose, to prevent a runny nose and soreness.

Effective remedy for Catarrh

Make sure that the sleeping room is well ventilated in summer and winter by airing it for at least 3 hours in the winter. This non-muggy atmosphere will help in curing this problem.

Mix 1 teaspoon full of honey with 1 teaspoon full of onion juice. Eat 1 teaspoon of this mixture, twice a day. This is considered to be a preventive for coughs and colds, especially catarrh, in winter.

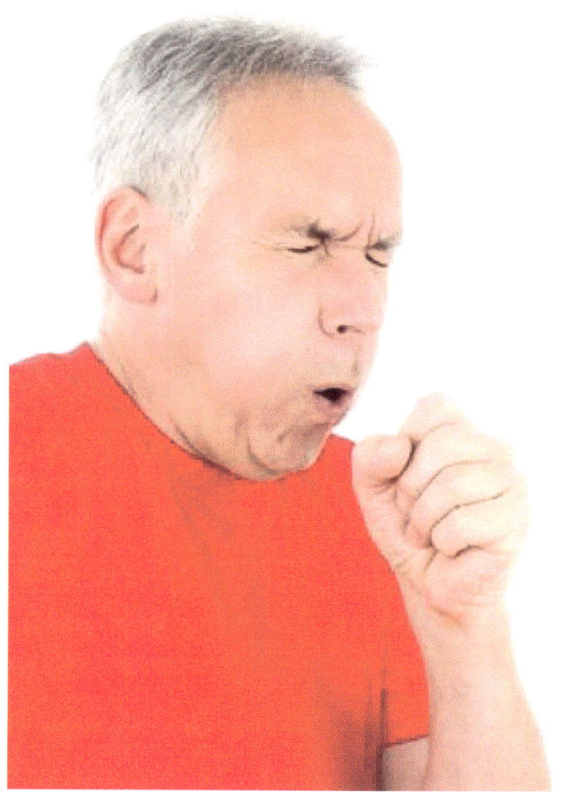

If you find your throat blocked with mucus, chew a clove with a little bit of sea salt sprinkled on it. This relieves any sort of irritation in your throat, and as the salt is an antiseptic, you are not going to suffer from any other infection in your throat. The clove has clove oil in it, and it is going to help cure your infection.

Breathing Problems

Mixed 1 teaspoon of camphor in half a cup of slightly warmed coconut oil and apply on the chest. This is going to help ease any sort of breathing problems.

A dry cough, especially if it is chronic can be removed if you eat plenty of red sweet apples for a week. This proves the adage, an Apple a day keeps the Doctor away. In the same manner, apples a week, keep cough and other such infections away.

Blocked nose

Make a saltwater solution with ¼ teaspoon of salt water in one glass of warm water. Sniff it gently to loosen all the accumulated mucus in your nasal passage. In fact, I gargle with this saltwater solution too, to prevent any throat infections in the winter. This remedy will be found very effective in catarrh because it loosens up the infected secretions and eliminates them. This also has an antiseptic action on your system.

Amazing Hay Fever remedy

Well, this remedy was found through sheer good luck and chance. A Canadian friend of mine suffering from hay fever was making coffee with real beans. She sneezed and accidentally dropped the coffee powder onto the lit kitchen stove. Well, the beans were well roasted and toasted, and the aroma of the coffee burnin' went straight up her nose. By the time the atmosphere was cleared up, 5 minutes or so, she found her hay fever had disappeared.

I was there to see it. I was coughing and sneezing along with her, [I do not like strong coffee fumes] but her hay-fever symptoms vanished like a bad nightmare. That means any of the irritating grains causing this allergy in her nostrils had been removed during the ensuing inhalation of coffee fumes and resulting sniffing and sneezing. Try this out right now, **guaranteed effective**, especially if you drink real coffee made from real coffee beans.

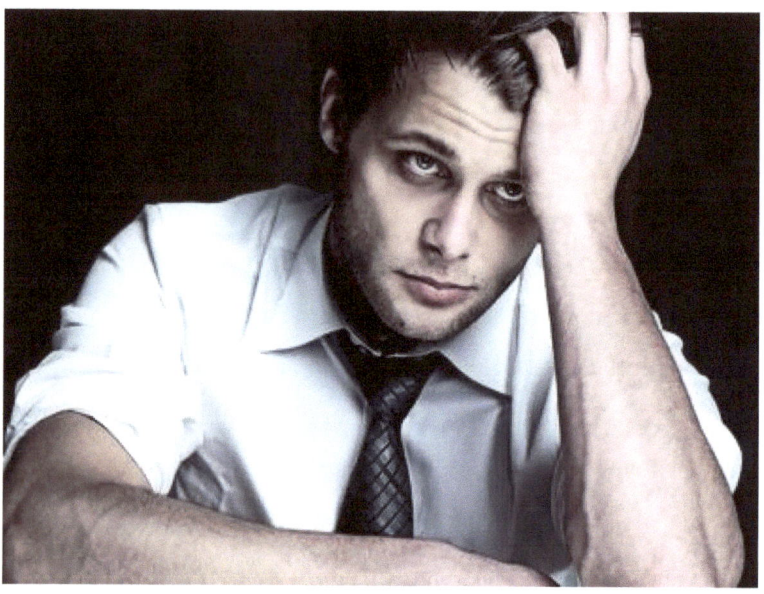

Suffering from Hay fever may make you feel run down.

If you are a regular sufferer of hay fever during the spring or autumn, try a change of climate, which is frequently quite beneficial. Some are relieved in the dry mountain air, while others are more benefited by the seashore or an ocean trip.

Look at this amazing way to **stop a nosebleed.**

The next time somebody suffers a nosebleed in your presence, dip a piece of white paper in water and put it under the upper lip. Now , have the patient press the upper lip with his fingers. Or you can press the end of the nose firmly against the partition between the nostrils. The scientific explanation is very easy. The patient is pressing an artery, and stopping the nose from bleeding anymore. You can also stop a nosebleed by placing a finger tight against the side of the nose for 15 minutes. This is going to stop the blood circulation and helps to form a blood clot.

Sore Throats

Believe it or not, this is the best way to get rid of sore throats.

Put cold packs on the throat. Gargle with very hot water and a little soda. This gets rid of the sore throat, overnight

Hoarseness – recipe for children

Take the juice of one lemon and saturate with honey, take a teaspoonful several times a day. Children love honey and they are going to drink this with pleasure.

Hoarseness – recipe for adults

Beat the white of one egg, juice of one lemon, with honey enough to thicken. Add one teaspoonful olive oil. Take one teaspoonful every hour until relieved. This is really effective I used this remedy, once before I had to go for a talk on stage, and apart from the stage fright, it was as if I had this creaking rusty piece of machinery in my throat, where once there was a larynx and a sound box. I started this remedy 30 hours before my talk and the hoarseness vanished.

Also, if you do not have to go outside, you can eat plenty of horseradish. This is supposed to be the best natural cure for hoarseness of your throat, even though it smells a bit too strong.

Grandma's natural cure for obesity

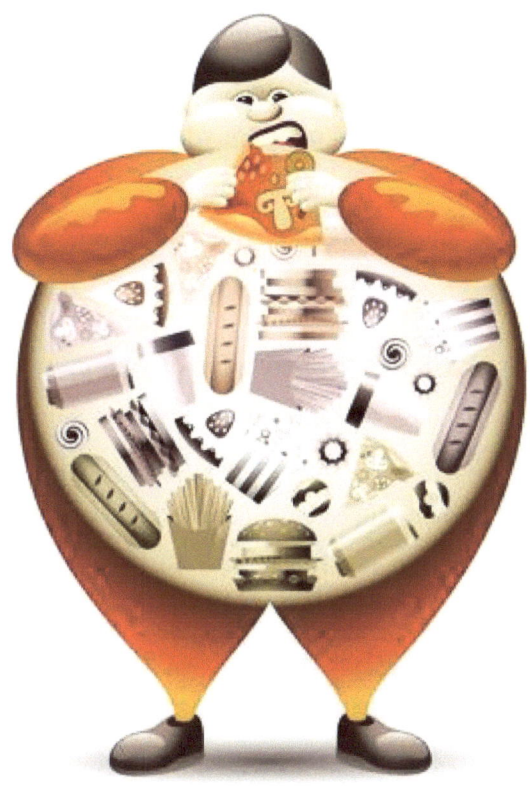

Grandma is definitely going to be annoyed if she looks down on us and sees how the generations following her are suffering from obesity or an excessive development of fat. Obesity may be headed a tree, which means that if your grandparents were fat, you are going to be fat and cannot have the silhouetted stick thin figure of Cindy Crawford. Obesity occurs most frequently in women of middle age, and also in children. Its chief causes excessive eating and drinking, especially of starchy and sugary foods.

Men grow fat, when they drink plenty of good malt liquors, including whiskey and beer. Our sedentary lifestyle is also one of the great factors contributing to so much weight around our waist regions and thigh regions. Lack of exercise may also cause you to grow fat. Remember that you need a little bit of fat in your food, to make your system work properly. That is the reason why cutting out fat altogether from your diet is not advisable. Your audio immune system is also going to be affected negatively, if you are fat. People suffering from obesity are more prone to autoimmune diseases like cardiovascular diseases, and other such problems.

Grandma would have advised the regulation of your diet, but that is so difficult for all of us. We love to eat and drink so much, and in such large quantities. Nevertheless, excess in food and drink, starchy foods and sugary foods foremost should be reduced considerably. Massages are supposed to help to break down the fat deposits. Start exercising.

Grandma's diet for Obesity

This is the diet which is normally recommended by dietitians and also by grandma, which is going to help reduce the fat content in your body. Remember that the weight loss has to be done slowly and steadily. Once your weight has reached the goal recommended to you by your doctor, you can continue with this diet to keep this weight steady.

Vegetables and fruit are recommended by doctors to start a regular and continuous weight loss.

For **breakfast,** you are going to have –

One or two cups of coffee or tea, without milk or sugar, but sweetened with a fraction of a grain of saccharin or artificial sweetener.

Three ounces of toasted or ordinary white bread or six ounces of brown bread; enough butter may be used to make the bread palatable – not more than one ounce.

Sliced raw tomatoes with vinegar, or cooked tomatoes without any sugar or fats.

This diet may be varied by the use of salted or fresh fish, either at breakfast or dinner. This fish must not be rich like salmon or sword-fish, but rather like perch or other small fish.

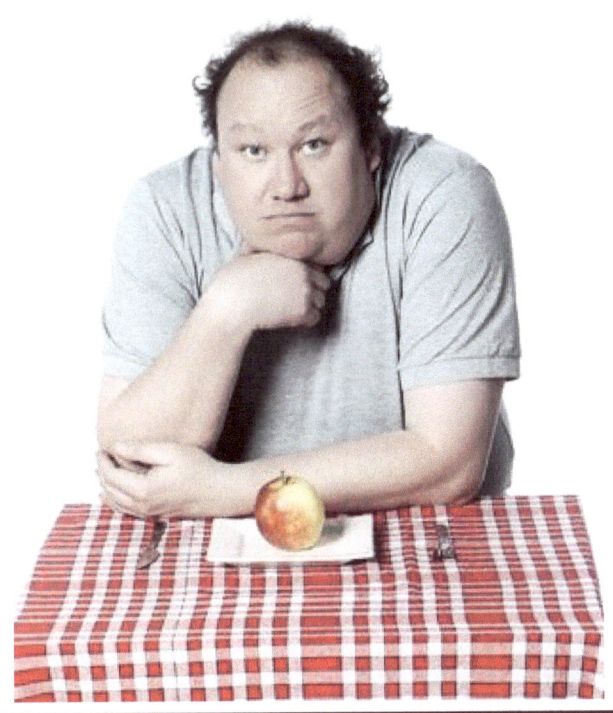

Noon Meal -

Soup, which can either be consommé or bouillon – without any cream, followed by a couple of pieces – white meat from poultry.

You may want to supplement the diet with stewed green vegetables, any sort, and little pieces of meat so that the dieter can get proper proteins.

As a salad, lettuce with olive oil, as well as vinegar mixed with citrus fruits like lemons, oranges, grapes, etc. are going to give the dieter his vitamins C. If he drinks coffee and tea, give it black without sugar and milk.

Dinner -

Dinner can be of one or two soft boiled eggs, – poached, but not fried – a few ounces of brown bread, some salad and fruit. I would rather prefer he drinks fresh fruit juice, instead of drinking tea and coffee before or after his meal. Prevent constipation by eating fiber rich fruit.

Before Going to Bed.--To prevent night starvation the patient may take a meal of biscuits and a little piece of cheese.

The reduction of the diet is generally best accomplished slowly and should be accompanied by measures devoted to the utilization of the fat present for the support of the body. Thus, the patient should not be too heavily clothed, either in the day or at night. He should also exercise daily. Make sure that the body is not dehydrated, by drinking lots of water.

Since ancient times, baths of the proper kind, cold, mustard or Turkish, has been used to get rid of extra fat, if the patient stands them well. No wonder spas are so popular to get rid of that extra fat.

Conclusion – and some general gossip!

I hope you liked volume 3 of grandma's natural remedies and ancient recipes. Grandma's recipes are natural, and have passed the test of time. There is absolutely no question of their ever having harmful side effects, unless of course you are using her dieting plan. The only harmful side effect is that you are going to crave food for the 1st week until your system gets used to lesser quantities of food.

Okay, let me admit it. I went on a diet, just once in my life, to see the scientific effect it would have on my physical, mental and emotional well-being. That was the scientific reason. The not so altruistic reason was that there was a party coming up and I needed to get rid of around 3 kgs real fast. This Israeli army diet was told to me by an army friend, who said that in his army it was necessary for army officers to maintain a steady weight of 72 kg. I still do not know whether Ari was pulling my leg or not.

This Israeli army diet is for 6 days. For the 1st 2 days, you just eat apples and nothing but apples. No tea no coffee, no liquid, except Apple juice. For the next 2 days, you eat nothing but cheese. Basically I love cheddar cheese, but I had reached the stage when I could not bear the thought of eating cheese after 2 days of cheese hunks and slices, with not even 2 hefty pieces of bread wrapped around them. Drink – plain water. The next 2 days – boiled chicken and nothing but boiled chicken.

Well, I dropped 4 kgs, and managed to fit in into my outfit. And believe me, I took double and triple helpings of everything on the overburdened buffet table, because I was so starved!

Did you notice that I did not eat greens, cereals and other food groups, – which would give me essential minerals – in my diet routine? The end result was that it took me 3 months to get my diet induced state of grouchiness , bad temper and touchiness back to my normal state of supposedly tranquil equanimity.

So remember, that a diet means you do not stop eating some food of a particular group, just because Beyoncé recommends it. The poor girl will take anywhere between 3 to 4 years to get back to her state of normal health, after she went on that terrible detoxification diet. This is also the reason why so many superstar actresses and models are so short tempered. They are not eating enough and they are not eating well.

Look out for more grandma's herbal remedies, recipes, cures and ways to keep healthy, naturally. Remember that grandma was a wise old woman. She tested out these remedies on her children, who naturally forgot how to collect them. But luckily, many of her recipes and remedies have survived and they are slowly and steadily being collected by people interested in natural cures like I.

You may want to know my credentials for writing remedies for curing diseases, which have no scientific and allopathic Degree behind me. Yes, I am not a qualified doctor, but since childhood, I have been living in areas where these natural remedies and recipes were used down the ages to survive in mountains and forests, far away from medical aid. I also learned about herbs from white witch doctors and herbalists, who would be called quacks or shamans by any experienced medical or scientific fraternity. They believed in alternative medicine passed down, down the ages from their ancestors. And these remedies worked.

That is why I grew up with a firm resolve never to indulge in drugs and pills while using natural ways in order to keep me and my family healthy.

So am I healthy, you may ask? Well, I have never been to a doctor since 1989 when I was in my early 20s. That was when I met with a potentially life-threatening accident and had to be hospitalized for 3 months. That was the first time since childhood, when I regularly used to go to the doctor to get my ears cleaned of a fungal infection. [*Otitis externa brought about by living in a moist mountainous climate and swimming in the rainwater-filled swimming pool in our garden.*]

The amount of chemical drugs they shoved into me to save me, helped me to survive and got rid of all the infections but it spoiled a system free of medicines so much that it took me about 5 years to get back to normal.

The doctors were more interested in making sure that my body survived. They were not much bothered about the harmful side effects such a heavy dosage of drugs- high dosage of antibiotics 3 times a day for 3 months – would have on a young otherwise healthy person, mentally, physically and psychologically. Nevertheless, I survived. And now I do not take any chemical-based Pills, vitamins, or any natural food supplements in pill form. All the medicines I use are topical – external natural remedies, especially Vaseline- camphor to prevent colds. These are medicines. I make myself out of time-tested remedies.

The end result is that I do not suffer from chronic diseases, autoimmune diseases or any other diseases, which may have occurred due to the harmful side effect of a long drug treatment. So now can you understand why I do not advocate going to a doctor for every small wound or scratch? QED.

This book is a grateful thanks to all those grandmothers out there along with the ancients, who passed on their knowledge to those who see and those who seek in the 21st century. So keep healthy and keep fit with grandma's natural remedies and ancient herbal tips. Grandma is going to be there to help you keep healthy, naturally, with her wise saws, economical tips and easy to utilize techniques which you can incorporate in your lifestyle right now!

Look out for more of grandma's natural remedies and herbal recipe volumes!

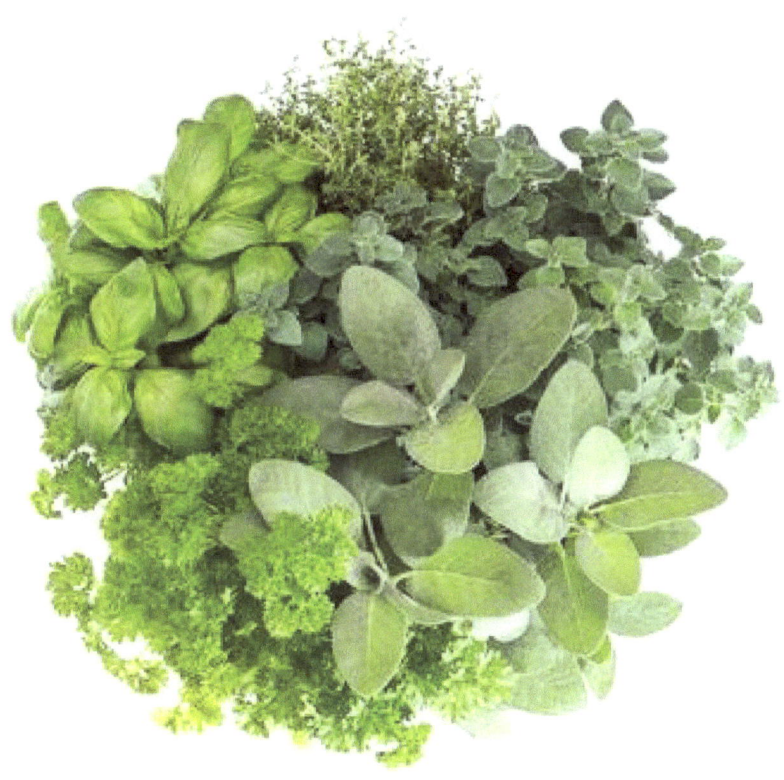

Author Bio

Dueep Jyot Singh is a Management and IT Professional who managed to gather Postgraduate qualifications in Management and English and Degrees in Science, French and Education while pursuing different enjoyable career options like being an hospital administrator, IT,SEO and HRD Database Manager/ trainer, movie scriptwriter, theatre artiste and public speaker, lecturer in French, Marketing and Advertising, ex-Editor of Hearts On Fire (now known as Solstice) Books Missouri USA, advice columnist and cartoonist, publisher and Aviation School trainer, ex- moderator on Medico.in, banker, student councilor ,travelogue writer … among other things! One fine morning, she decided that she had enough of killing herself by Degrees and went back to her first love -- writing. It is more enjoyable! She already has 48 published academic and 14 fiction- in- different- genre books under her belt.

When she is not designing websites or making Graphic design illustrations for clients, she is busy browsing in old bookshops for antique books and 1st editions, or just pottering around the forests and mountains for a bit of exploring, collecting herbs and plants and trekking.

Check out some of the other JD-Biz Publishing books

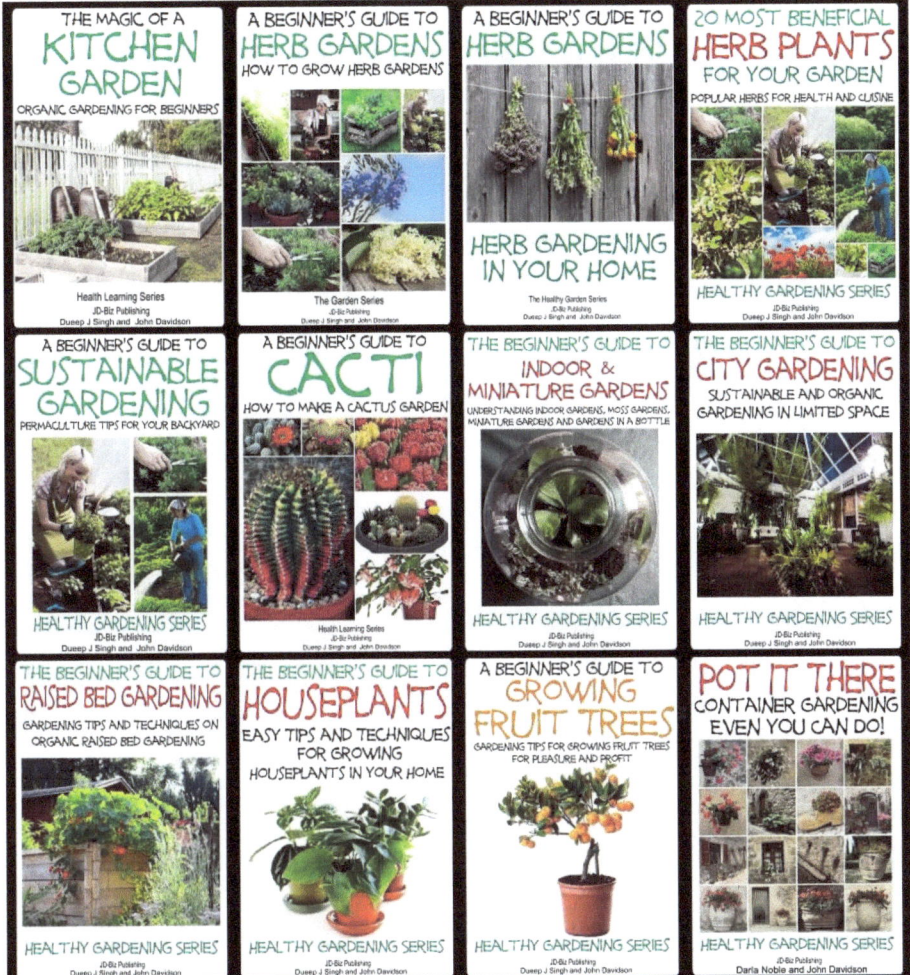

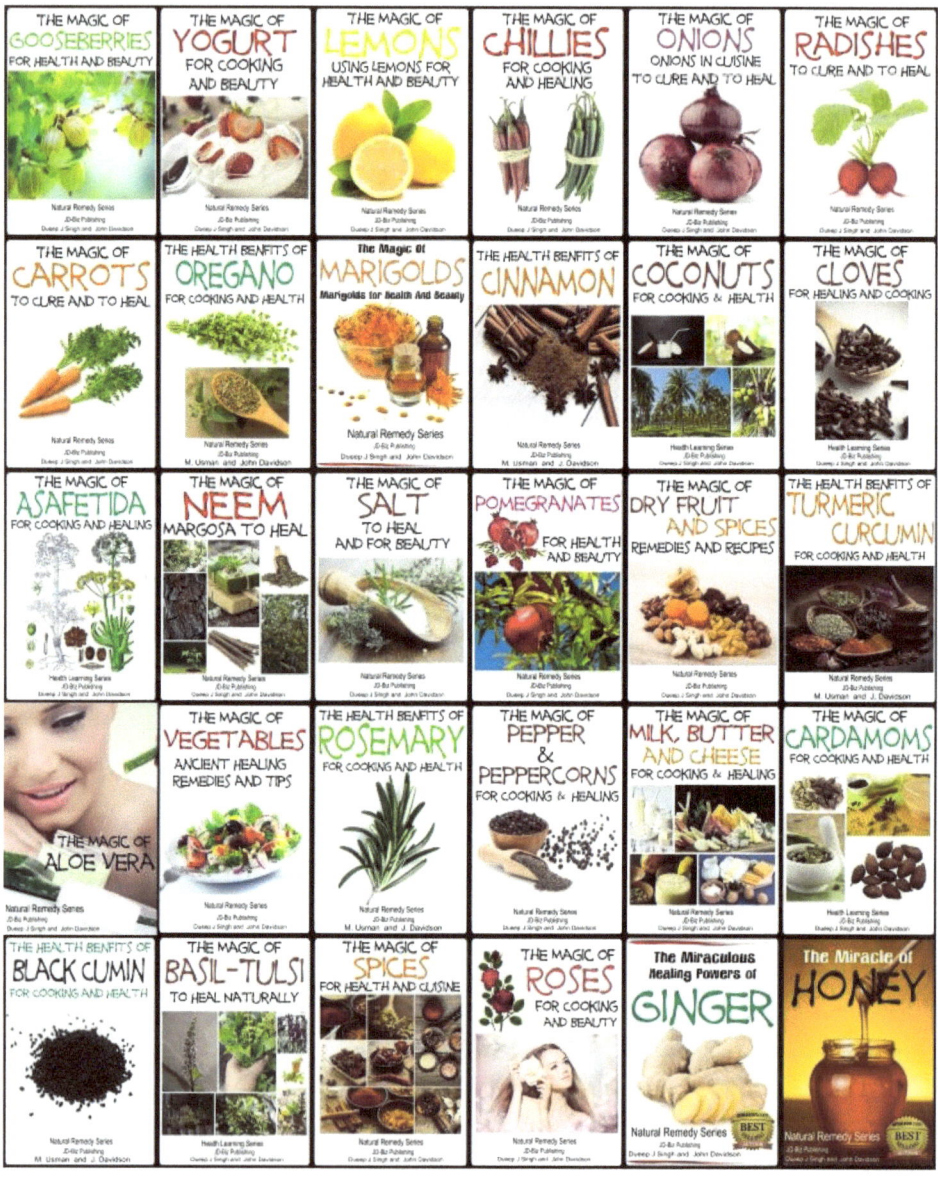

Country Life Books

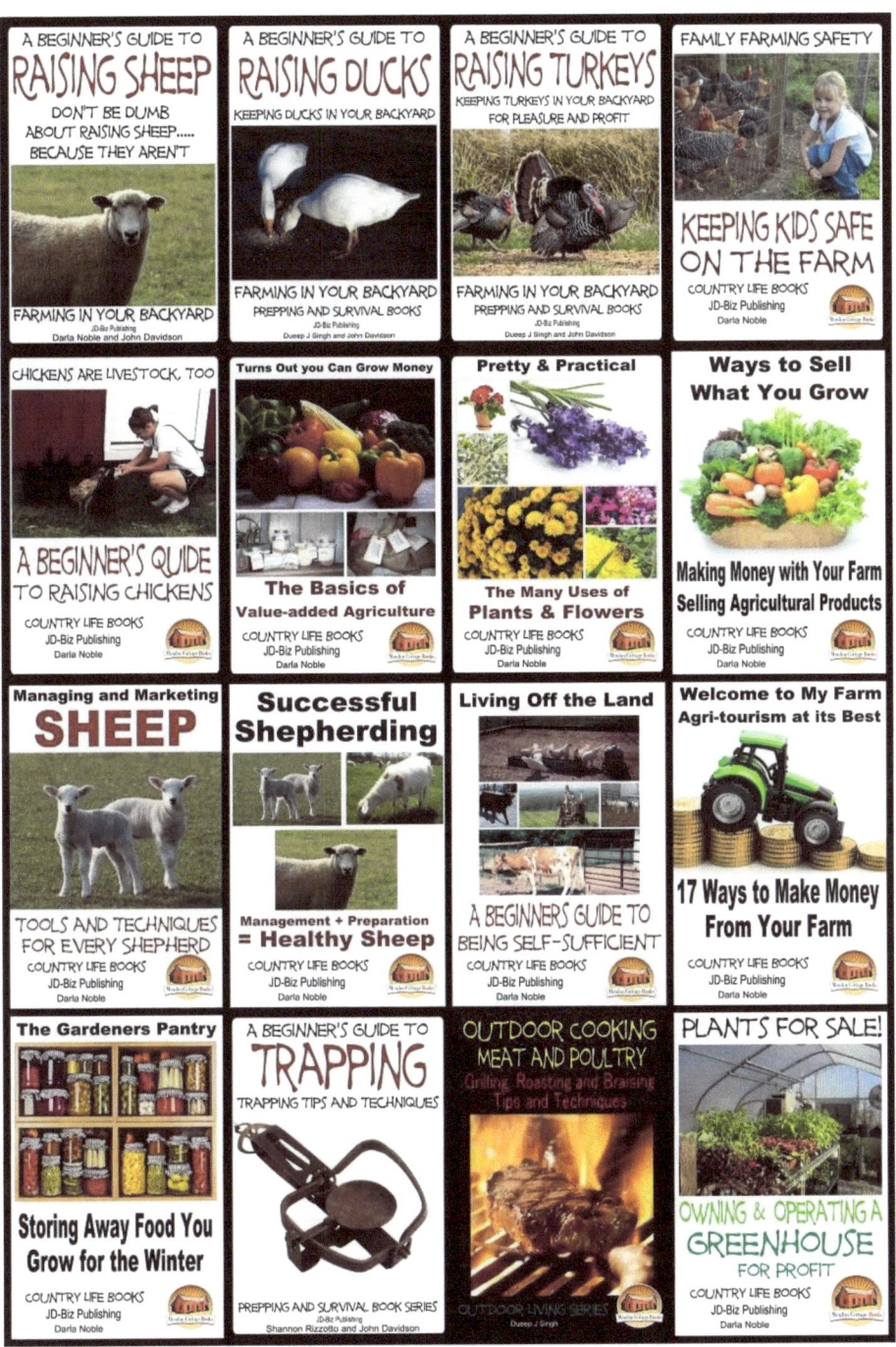

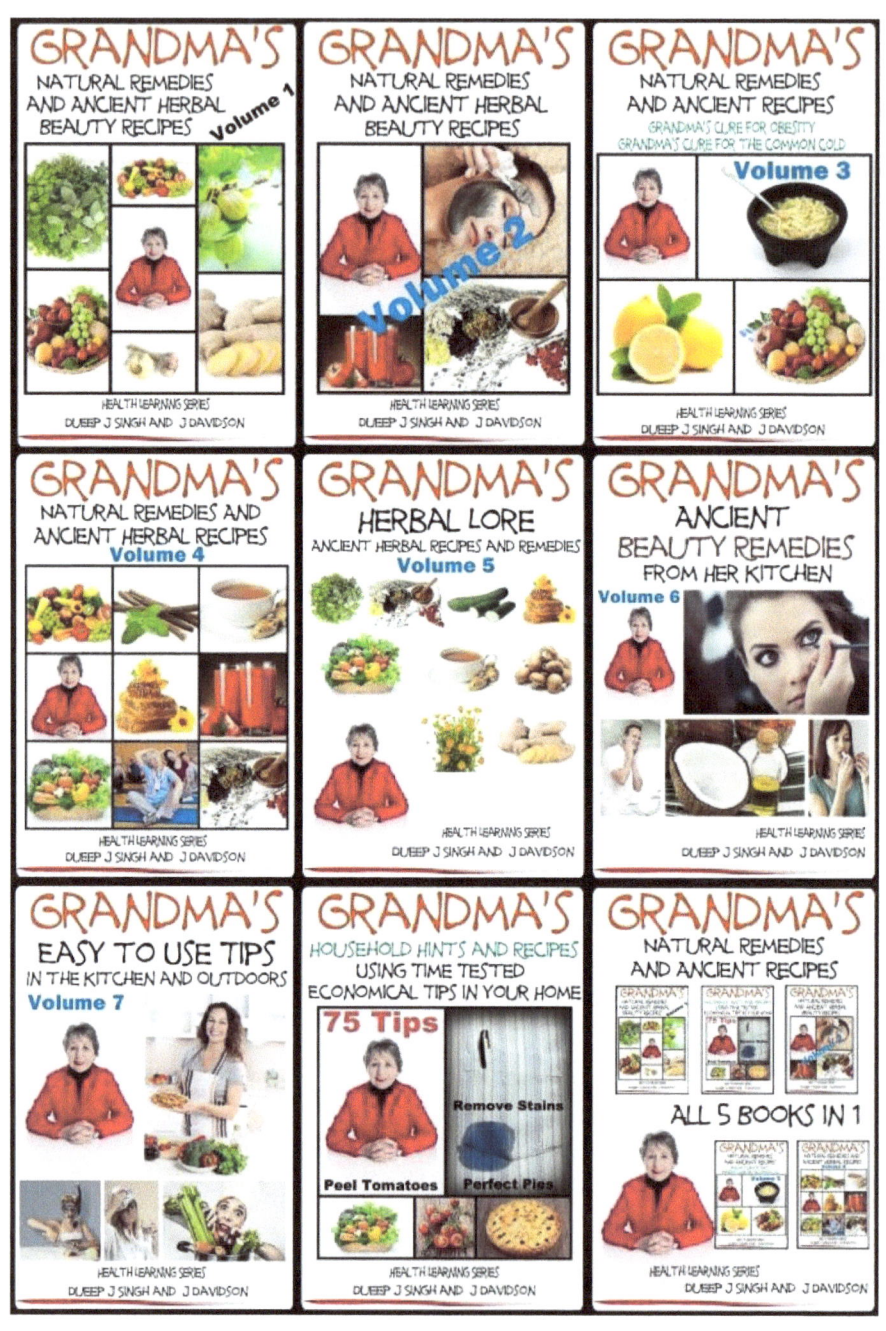

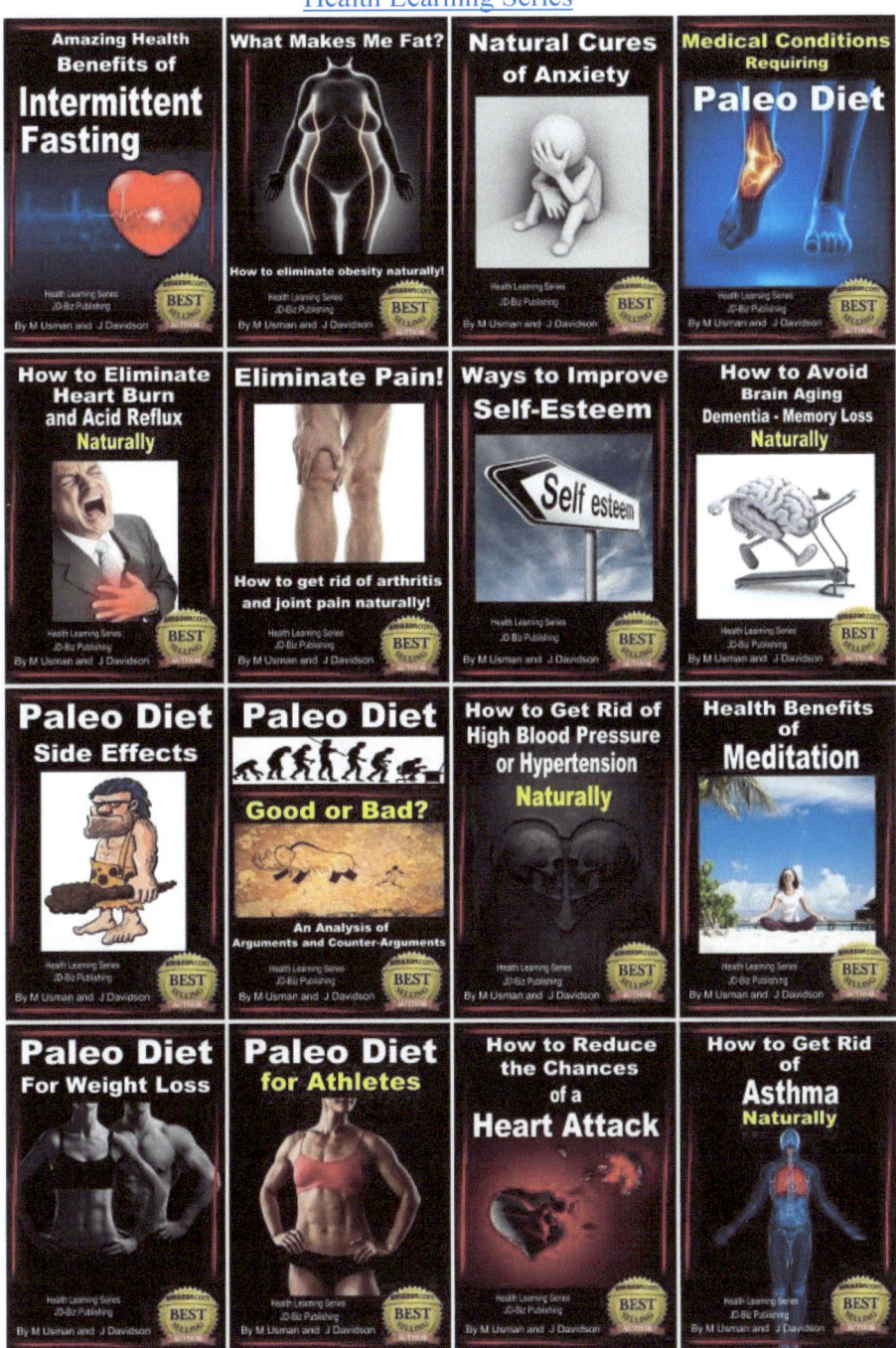

Amazing Animal Book Series

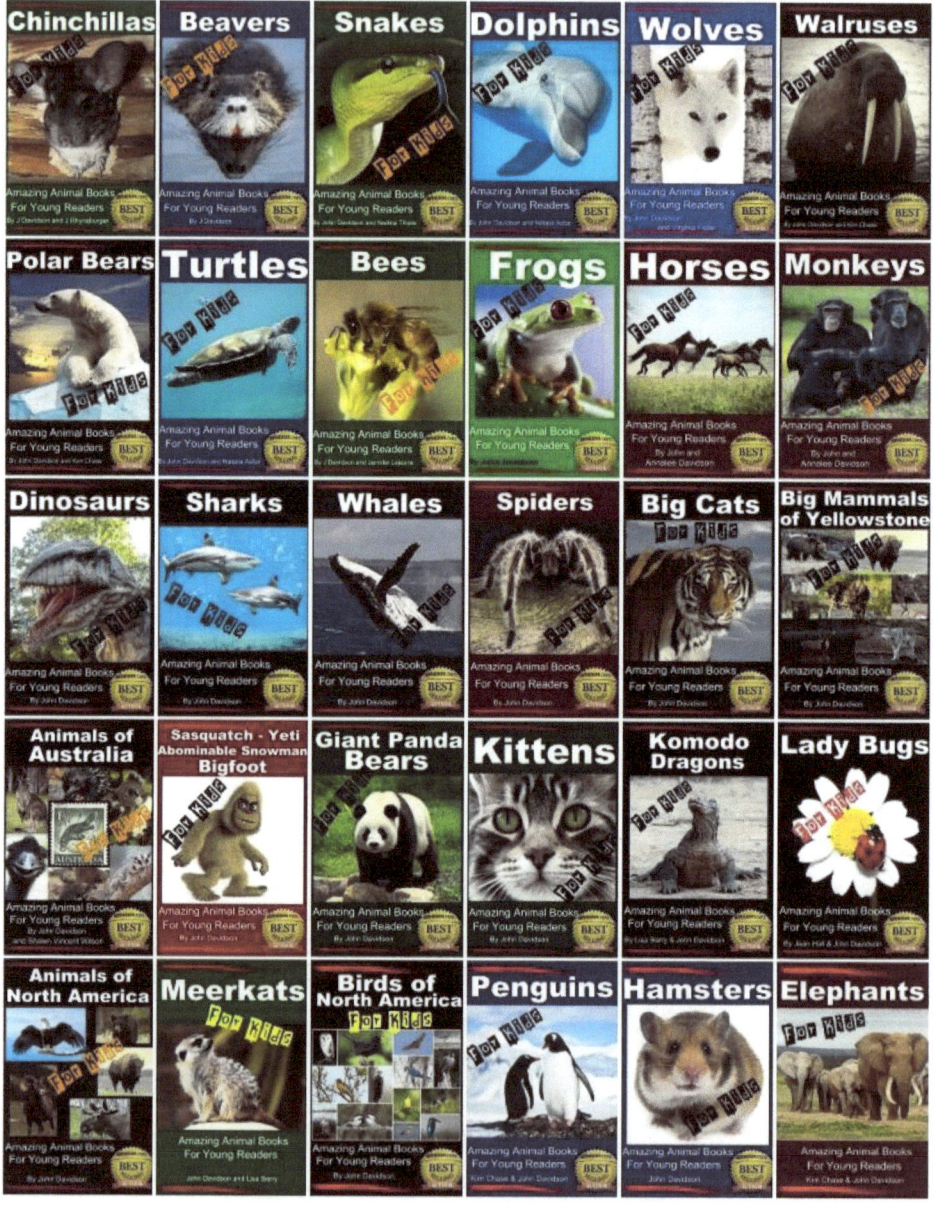

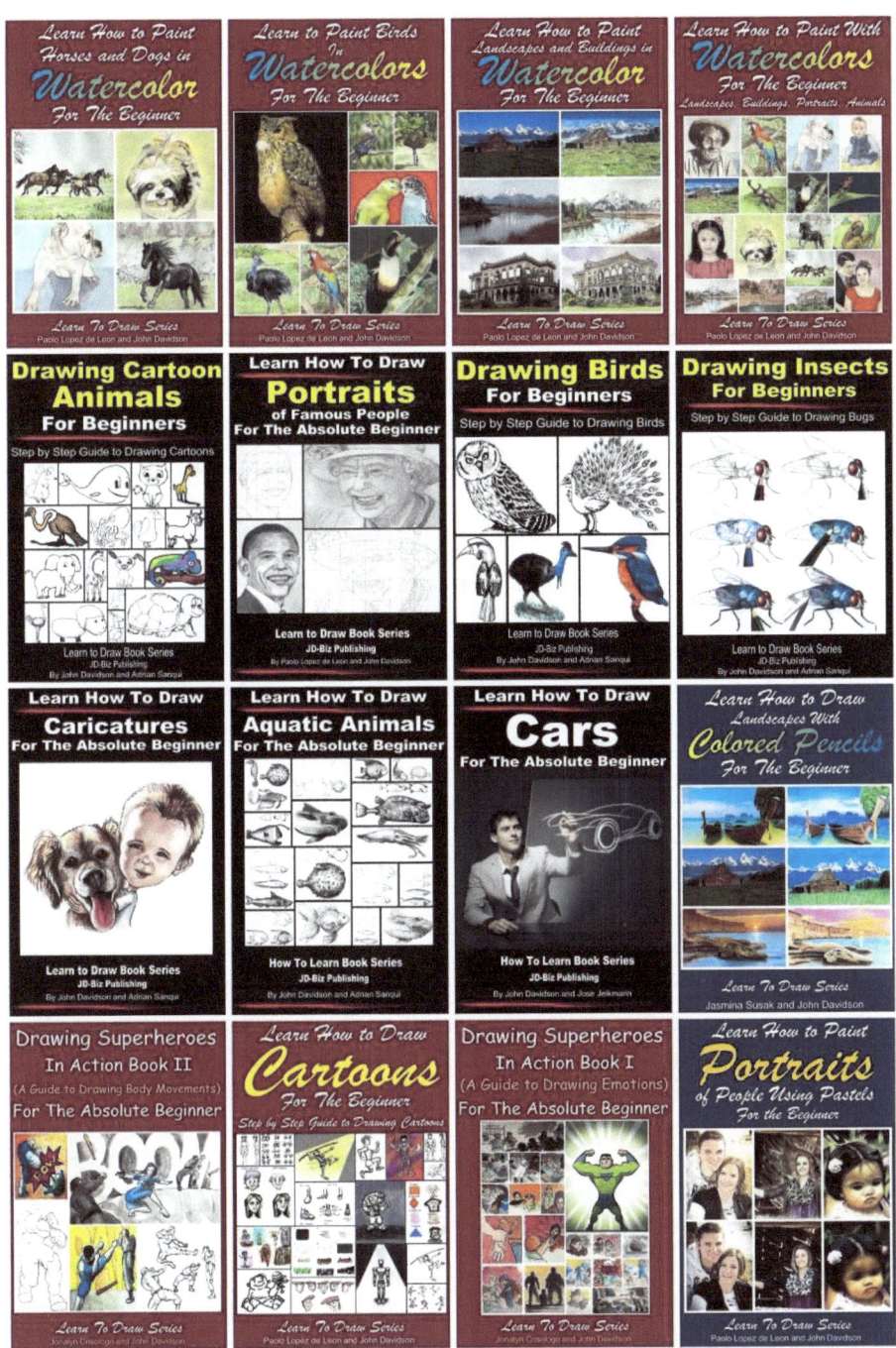

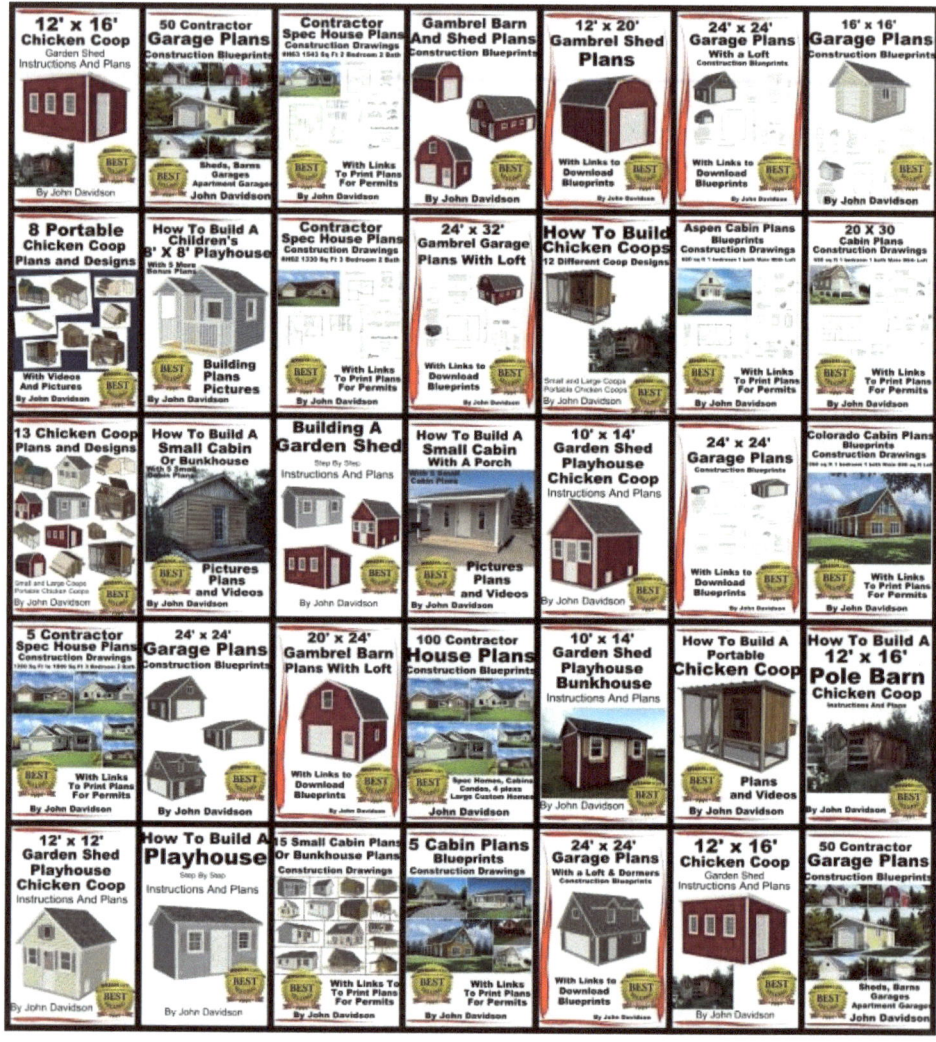

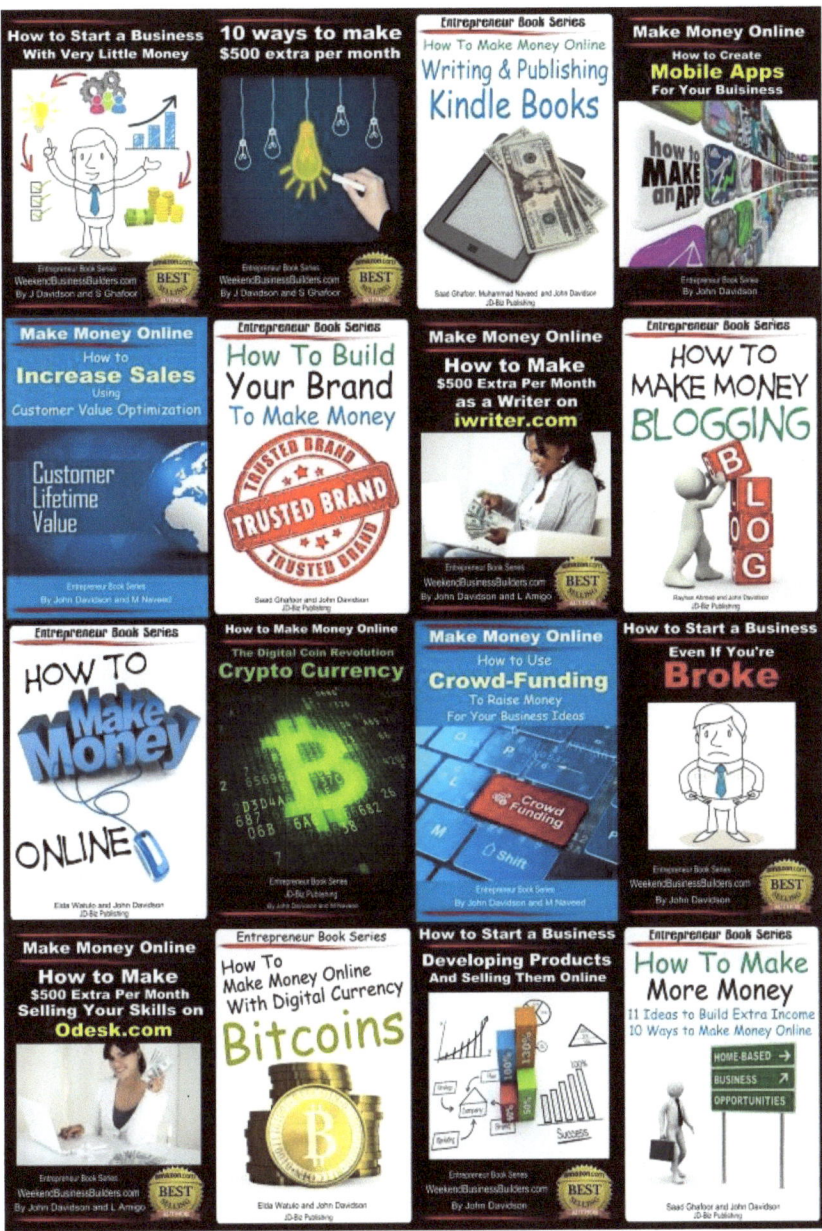

Our books are available at

1. Amazon.com

2. Barnes and Noble

3. Itunes

4. Kobo

5. Smashwords

6. Google Play Books

Download Free Books!

http://MendonCottageBooks.com

Publisher

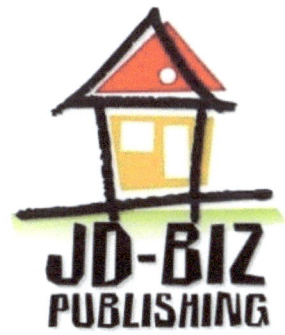

JD-Biz Corp

P O Box 374

Mendon, Utah 84325

http://www.jd-biz.com/

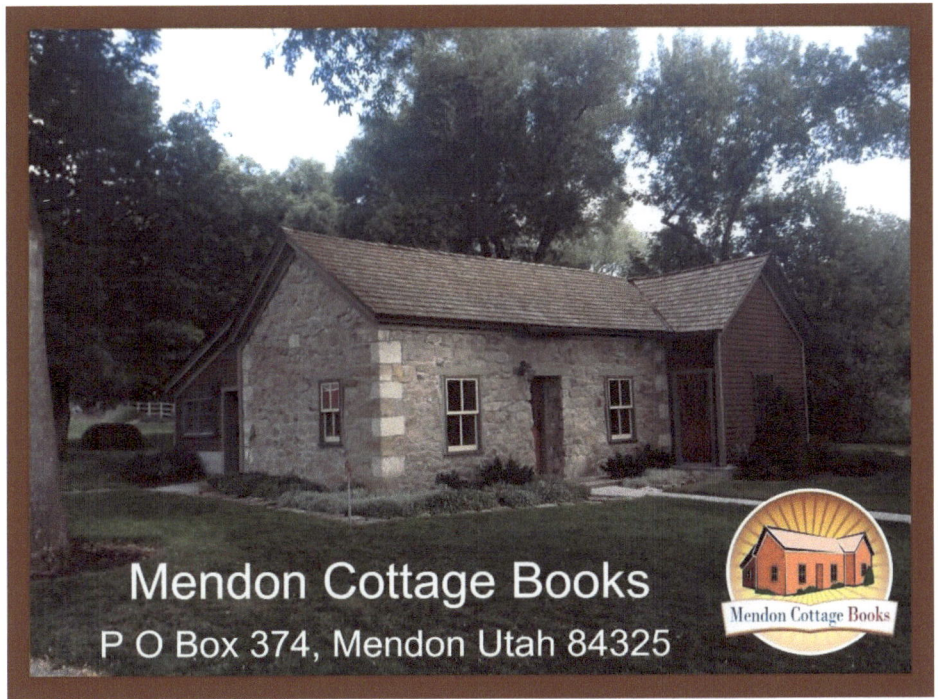